- Clinical Nutrition -

A PRACTICAL GUIDE TO DIABETES NUTRITION

Practical Guide for Nutritionists

FIRST EDITION

Dr. Amin Gasmi

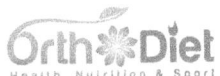

© Copyright 2020 by Dr. Amin Gasmi - All rights reserved.

The contents of this book may not be reproduced, duplicated or transmitted without direct written permission from the author.

Under no circumstances will any legal responsibility or blame be held against the publisher for any reparation, damages, or monetary loss due to the information herein, either directly or indirectly.

Legal Notice:

This book is copyright protected. This is only for personal use. You cannot amend, distribute, sell, use, quote or paraphrase any part or the content within this book without the consent of the author.

Disclaimer Notice:

Please note the information contained within this document is for educational and entertainment purposes only. Every attempt has been made to provide accurate, up to date and reliable complete information. No warranties of any kind are expressed or implied. Readers acknowledge that the author is not engaging in the rendering of legal, financial, medical or professional advice. The content of this book has been derived from various sources. Please consult a licensed professional before attempting any techniques outlined in this book.

By reading this document, the reader agrees that under no circumstances is the author responsible for any losses, direct or indirect, which are incurred as a result of the use of information contained within this document, including, but not limited to, —errors, omissions, or inaccuracies.

DEDICATION

To the ultimate power of the universe, the power of love. For me, more than all: dad, mom, my wife, Alain, Cherif and Salva.

ACKNOWLEDGEMENT

I thank all those who throughout my life have contributed to my training and make me what I have become today: God, my family, my teachers, my colleagues, my friends, my students, my patients, my athletes, and everyone I have met on my way. I am also indebted to a large number of books and scientific articles, and I cannot thank their authors enough for their sharing and generosity.

TABLE OF CONTENTS

Dedication iii

Acknowledgement iv

1.0: Introduction 1

2.0: Role of diet therapy in the treatment of diabetes 3

3.0: Goals of diet therapy in diabetes 4

4.0: Principles of diet therapy in diabetes 6

    4.1   Carbohydrate intake in diabetes 6

    4.2   Dietary fibers intake in sugar diabetes 14

    4.3   Use of sweeteners in diabetes 14

    4.4   Fat intake in diabetes 20

    4.5   Protein intake in diabetes 21

    4.6   Vitamins and minerals in diabetes 22

    4.7   Fluid intake in diabetes 23

    4.8   Energy value of the diet in diabetes patient 24

5.0: Diet therapy for diabetes 25

    5.1   General dietary requirements for diabetes 25

    5.2   Diet Therapy Tactics for Diabetes 26

    5.3   Features of diet therapy for patients receiving insulin 28

    5.4   Diet therapy for patients with a threat of diabetic coma . 30

    5.5   Diet therapy for possible hypoglycemia 31

    5.6   Diabetes Prevention.. 32

6.0: Phytotherapy for diabetes 34

    6.1   Recommendations for the use of medicinal plants for diabetes.. 34

7.0: Type of diet used for the treatment of diabetes.................... 37

    7.1   Diabetes Diet... 37

    7.2   Trial diet 43

    7.3   Insulin diet... 44

    7.4   Option Diabetes Diet for patients with bronchial asthma 45

    7.5   High Protein Diet.. 56

    7.6   Main option for a standard diet... 57

    7.7   Low-calorie standard diet option (low-calorie diet).......... 59

Author's presentation... 61

References 62

INTRODUCTION

In 2002, experts from the American Diabetes Association carried out a technical review of the results of various randomized and controlled trials over the past 8 years. These studies have made it possible to formulate principles and recommendations for the management and prevention of sugar diabetes.

The goals of the recommendations were to improve the quality of treatment and the life of patients with diabetes mellitus - life with diabetes, not diabetes.

The treatment of diabetes mellitus of any type is complex and includes diet, dosed physical activity, training of patients with diabetes self-control, drug therapy, prevention and treatment of late complications.

In the treatment of all types of diabetes, it is necessary to strive for normal indicators of daily fluctuations in blood sugar. The main indicators indicating the state of compensation in diabetes mellitus are normal values of fasting blood glucose and during the day, as well as the absence of glucose in the urine.

Clinical nutrition is an integral component of diabetes treatment and an indispensable part of the self-training of patients. The main principle of dietary nutrition for diabetes is the focus on the normalization of metabolic disorders.

Nutrition recommendations should be based not only on scientific approaches but also take into account the changing lifestyle, activity of life positions, physical activity, cultural and ethnic preferences of patients. It is necessary to constantly monitor the level of glycemia, lipids, blood pressure, as their increase increases the risk of various complications of diabetes.

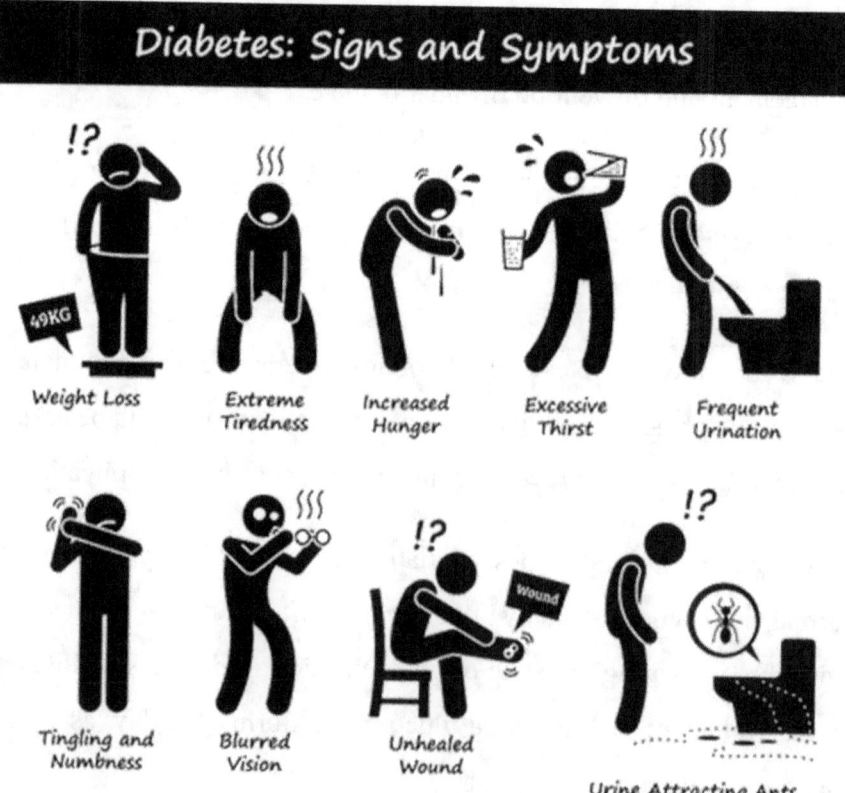

ROLE OF DIET THERAPY IN THE TREATMENT OF DIABETES

In the past (before the use of insulin and oral hypoglycemic drugs), diet was almost the only way to treat diabetes.

With the experience of using insulin and oral hypoglycemic drugs in the treatment of patients with diabetes mellitus, the attitude towards diet therapy has gradually changed. In some countries, endocrinologists began to practice the so-called free diet (nutrition without any restrictions), based on monitoring the patient's condition with insulin or drugs that increase insulin in the blood plasma. In this case, improper selection of the dose of insulin led to an increase in glycemia, body weight, an increase in insulin doses due to the development of resistance to it, and the progression of complications of diabetes.

Currently, around the world, diet therapy for patients with diabetes is receiving much attention.

GOALS OF DIET THERAPY IN DIABETES

According to the recommendations of the American Diabetes Association in 2002, the main goals of diet therapy for diabetes are as follows:

1. Achieving and maintaining metabolic processes at an optimal level.

   - Achieving normal fluctuations in blood glucose levels or bringing them as close as possible to normal levels to prevent or reduce possible risks of complications.

   - Normalize lipid metabolism to reduce the risk of macrovascular complications.

2. Maintaining normal blood pressure levels to reduce the risk of cardiovascular complications.

3. Prevention and treatment of diabetes complications; modification of food intake and lifestyle for the prevention and treatment of obesity, dyslipidemia, cardiovascular diseases, including arterial hypertension and nephropathy.

4. Use of "healthy" foods and physical activity to improve diabetes.

5. Food intake should take into account personal and cultural characteristics, lifestyle, patient wishes and willingness to change.

6. Patients of a young age with type I diabetes need to ensure adequate energy consumption of food to guarantee normal growth and development; comply with the regimen of insulin administration with food intake and physical activity.

7. Young patients with type II diabetes need to contribute to changes in eating behavior and physical activity to reduce insulin resistance.

8. Provide pregnant or lactating women with essential nutrients with adequate energy requirements for normal reproductive functions.

9. For older people, provide nutritional and psychosocial needs according to age.

10. For persons receiving treatment with insulin or insulin secretion enhancing drugs, organize training on self-treatment of hypoglycemia, acute diseases, glycemic disorders associated with physical activity.

11. To reduce the risk of developing diabetes in individuals predisposed to it, encourage physical activity, decrease in body weight if it is increased, or at least prevent its increase.

PRINCIPLES OF DIET THERAPY IN DIABETES

The main principle of the diet is to bring it as close as possible to the physiological norms of nutrition of a healthy person of the corresponding gender, age, height, physique, profession and physical activity, psychosocial and cultural wishes of the patient himself.

Diet therapy for patients with diabetes should be carried out taking into account the severity of the disease, the presence of complications, concomitant diseases.

4.1 Carbohydrate intake in diabetes

The main attention in the diet of patients with diabetes should be given to the carbohydrate part of the diet. Carbohydrates are a major energy provider. In rational nutrition, they account for 54–56% of the daily energy value of the diet, with diabetes - from 40 to 60%.

Complex carbohydrates (oligo- and polysaccharides) and simple (mono- and disaccharides) exist. Complex carbohydrates are divided into digestible in the gastrointestinal tract (starch, glycogen) and indigestible (cellulose, hemicellulose, pectin substances).

Historically, the most important principle of medical nutrition for patients with diabetes has been the exclusion from the diet of foods and dishes rich in easily digestible carbohydrates: sugar, honey, jam, chocolate, cakes, cookies, marmalade, as well as semolina and rice.

It should be remembered that these products can be used to stop sudden hypoglycemia, as well as in the treatment of ketoacidosis.

A severe restriction of sweets in the diet of some patients is not well tolerated psychologically. Therefore, the technique of "encouragement" is permissible when the patient occasionally allows himself to eat a usually forbidden product (for example, cake, candy). This technique allows the patient to feel like a full-fledged person and it is easier to follow a diet.

The diet of patients contains mainly complex carbohydrates: bread, cereals, vegetables, fruits, berries. In products of plant origin (especially fruits and berries), alkaline valencies predominate, which is very important for the fight against acidosis.

4.1.1 Classification of plant products and carbohydrate content

According to the carbohydrate content, vegetables, fruits, and berries are divided into three groups.

1. Fruits with 100 g of which contain less than 5 g of carbohydrates: cucumbers, tomatoes, white and cauliflower, zucchini, eggplant, lettuce, sorrel, spinach, rhubarb, radish, radish, mushrooms, pumpkin, dill, cranberries, lemons, sea

buckthorn, apples, and plum sour varieties. These foods can be consumed up to 600-800 g per day.

2. Vegetables, fruits and berries, 100 g of which contain from 5 to 10 g of carbohydrates: carrots, beets, onions, rutabaga, celery, sweet peppers, beans, tangerines, oranges, grapefruit, apricots, cherry plum, watermelon, melon, dogwood, pear , peaches, lingonberries, strawberries, raspberries, currants, gooseberries, blueberries, quinces, sweet varieties of apples and plums. They are recommended to consume up to 200 g per day.

3. Vegetables, fruits and berries, 100 g of which contain more than 10 g of carbohydrates: potatoes, green peas, sweet potatoes (sweet potato), pineapples, bananas, pomegranates, cherries, figs, dates, persimmons, cherries, aronia, grapes, dried fruits (raisins, figs, prunes, dried apricots). The use of these products is not recommended due to the rapid increase in blood glucose levels when they are absorbed. Potatoes are allowed in an amount of 200-300 g per day, taking into account the exact amount of carbohydrates.

4.1.2 Glycemic index

The glycemic index is an indicator that reflects the ability of food to increase blood sugar. High glycemic index foods provide a quick increase in blood sugar. They are easily digested and absorbed by the body. The higher the glycemic index of a particular product, the higher when it enters the body, the blood sugar level will rise, which, in turn, will entail the production of a powerful portion of insulin by the body. Foods with a low glycemic index raise blood sugar levels more slowly because the carbohydrates in these foods are not immediately absorbed. Determining the glycemic index of a product depends on many factors: the type of carbohydrate that the food contains, the amount of fiber contained in it, how long the product has been cooked, the presence of protein and fat in the product. The glycemic index is a relative concept. When compiling it, glucose was initially taken, its glycemic index was equal to 100, and the indices of all other products make up a certain amount of percent relative to the glycemic index of glucose. In some cases, white bread is not taken as a reference point for the glycemic index. Regarding the values of the glycemic index of glucose or white bread, the glycemic indices of all other products are calculated.

- The more fiber-containing foods in various foods, the lower the total glycemic index.

- Raw vegetables and fruits have a lower glycemic index than those cooked.

- The combination of proteins with carbohydrates reduces the overall glycemic index.

- The more the product is crushed, the higher its glycemic index.

- The longer the food is chewed, the slower the absorption of carbohydrates (the lower post-nutritional glycemia).

Glycemic Index

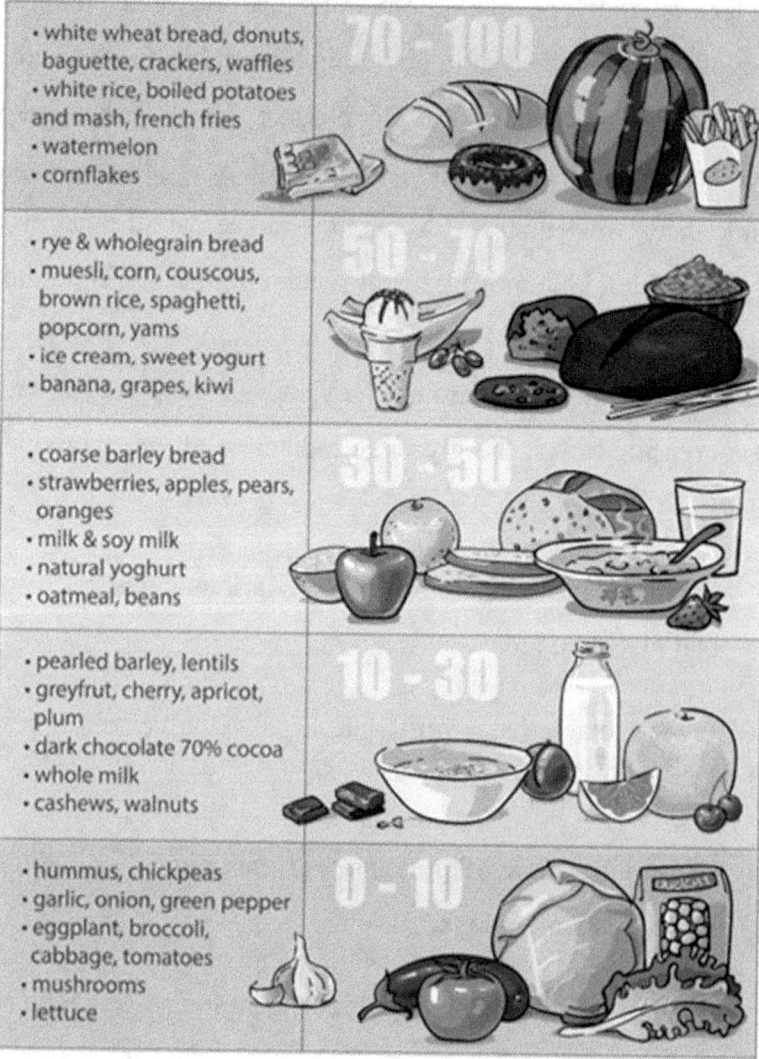

• white wheat bread, donuts, baguette, crackers, waffles • white rice, boiled potatoes and mash, french fries • watermelon • cornflakes	70 - 100
• rye & wholegrain bread • muesli, corn, couscous, brown rice, spaghetti, popcorn, yams • ice cream, sweet yogurt • banana, grapes, kiwi	50 - 70
• coarse barley bread • strawberries, apples, pears, oranges • milk & soy milk • natural yoghurt • oatmeal, beans	30 - 50
• pearled barley, lentils • greyfrut, cherry, apricot, plum • dark chocolate 70% cocoa • whole milk • cashews, walnuts	10 - 30
• hummus, chickpeas • garlic, onion, green pepper • eggplant, broccoli, cabbage, tomatoes • mushrooms • lettuce	0 - 10

4.1.3 Carbohydrate Interchangeability

In diabetes patients who are on a strict diet, the carbohydrate content in the daily diet should be constant. To diversify the menu, you need to know the rules for the interchangeability of products for carbohydrates.

For this purpose, the concept of "bread unit" (XE) is introduced.

4.1.3.1 What is a bread unit ?

1 XE - this is the amount of product that contains 12 g to 15 g of carbohydrates (corresponding to approximately 50 kcal). The processing of 1 XE requires approximately 2 PIECES of insulin. One meal should not be eaten more than 6-8 XE.

Initially, a bread unit was introduced specifically for patients with diabetes receiving insulin. They need to observe the daily intake of carbohydrates corresponding to the administered insulin. So, if you make a mistake in choosing foods and eat more carbohydrates than is calculated according to the prescribed dose of insulin, the blood sugar level will increase. Conversely, if you regularly get less carbohydrates than you need, you may develop hypoglycemia.

Thanks to the introduction of the concept of a bread unit, patients with diabetes got the opportunity to correctly compose a menu, competently replacing some carbohydrate-containing products with others.

The daily human need for carbohydrates is approximately 18-25 bread units. It is advisable to distribute them into six meals. At breakfast, lunch, and dinner, it is recommended to take 3-5 bread units of carbohydrates, in the second breakfast and afternoon snack - 1 bread unit. Most carbohydrate-containing foods should be in the morning.

Using the tables of the chemical composition of food products, you can calculate the bread units for any product. Thus, it is possible to diversify the carbohydrate part of the diet, but the total amount of carbohydrates will remain constant. For example, instead of a piece of rye bread weighing 50 g (2 XE), you can eat 300 g of blueberries (2 XE) or drink 0.5 l of milk (2 XE), or eat 150 g of boiled potatoes (2 XE).

4.1.3.2 Interchangeable Products

- Bakery and grain products. Equivalent: 40 g (slice) of wheat bread, 50 g of rye bread, 40 g of bakery products, 100 g of protein-wheat bread, 140 g of protein-bran bread, 30 g of crackers (2 pieces), 20 g of peas (beans).

- Products containing animal protein. Equivalent: 30 g of boiled beef, 50 g of veal, 65 g of lean pork, 48 g of chicken, 46 g of turkey, 46 g of rabbit, 77 g of cooked sausage, 85 g of sausages (sausages), 54 g of fish, 35 g of Dutch cheese, 53 g low-fat cottage cheese, 1.5 eggs.

- Fats. Equivalent: 5 g butter, 4 g ghee, 4 g vegetable oil, 40 g cream of 10% fat, 16 g sour cream, 6 g mayonnaise.

- Milk products. Equivalent: 200 g of kefir, 200 g of milk, 200 g of yogurt.

- Vegetables. Equivalent: 50 g of potatoes, 90 g of beets, 140 g of carrots, 170 g of turnips, 75 g of green peas.

- Fruits and berries. Equivalent: 100 g apples, 110 g apricots, 100 g cherries, 105 g pears, 115 g plums, 90 g cherries, 135 g orange, 140 g garden strawberries, 115 g gooseberries, 125 g raspberries, 130 g currants.

- The number of lemons and cranberries can be practically unlimited in the diet of patients with diabetes.

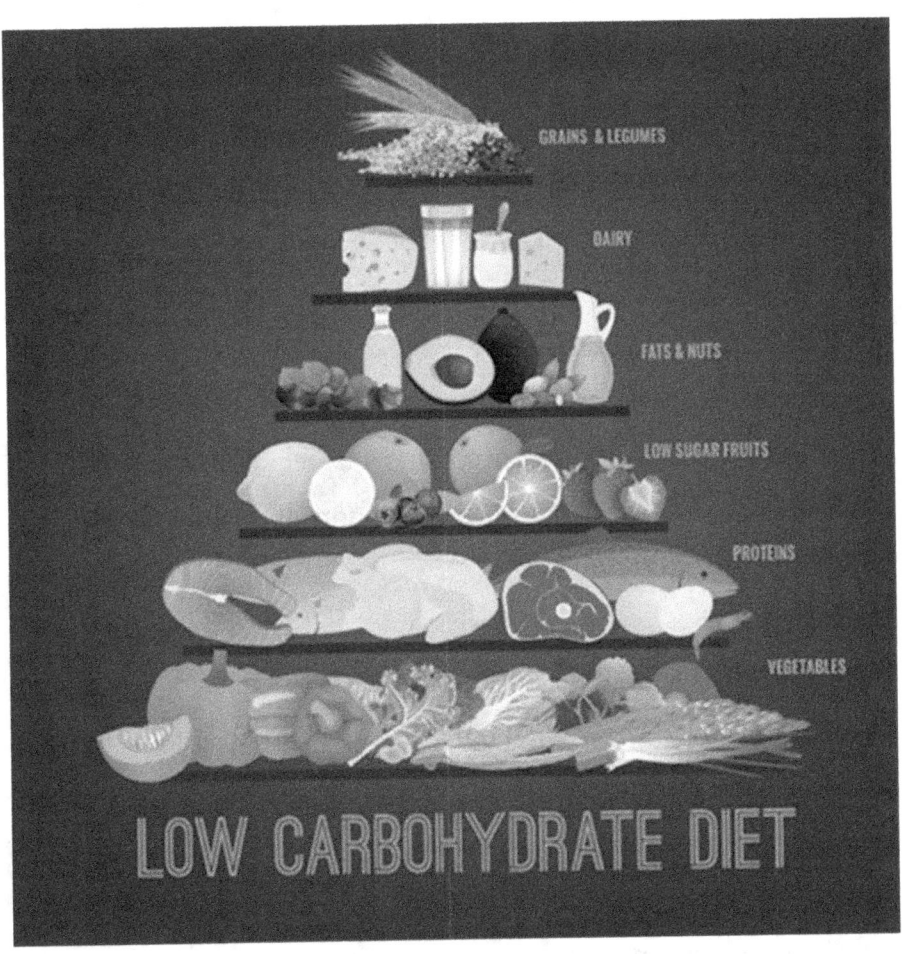

4.2 Dietary fibers intake in sugar diabetes

Scientists have long known the ability of plant-based products to lower blood sugar due to the presence of dietary fiber and hypoglycemic substances in them, many of which are guanidine derivatives.

Cabbage and Brussels sprouts have a sugar-lowering effect, grapefruits, lemons, oranges, onions, garlic, mushrooms, spinach, celery, oats, blueberries, strawberries. Recently, the attention of scientists has been attracted by Jerusalem artichoke (earthen pear), which contains insulin and has a sugar-lowering effect. Due to the presence of potassium, iron, silicon, and zinc, Jerusalem artichoke has a positive effect on electrolyte metabolism in diabetes mellitus.

In recent years, indigestible polysaccharides (cellulose, hemicellulose, pectin) have been given great importance in the diet therapy of diabetes mellitus. Dietary fiber stimulates intestinal motility, reduces the absorption of cholesterol and fatty acids, adsorb toxic products in the intestines, as well as some proteins, fats, and carbohydrates. The positive effect of dietary fiber, according to recent data, manifests itself when it is received in large quantities (more than 40-50 g per day, instead of 25-30 g).

4.3 Use of sweeteners in diabetes

The need to exclude or sharply limit the use of sugar in food creates a state of discomfort in patients with diabetes mellitus. Especially difficult for children and adolescents to tolerate the exclusion of sweets, so sugar substitutes obtained from plants or created chemically have found widespread use.

Patients can mainly use stevia extract, xylitol and to a lesser extent fructose as sugar substitutes. The other sweeteners should not be used frequently and regularly due to their potential side effects and to very few data regarding their safety for the human body.

4.3.1 General rules for the use of sweeteners

- It is necessary to establish individual intolerance to xylitol and sorbitol, taking into account their laxative effect.

- Take sweeteners only against the background of compensation or sum compensation of the disease.

- It is necessary to take into account the energy value of sweeteners.

- The daily dose of xylitol, sorbitol or fructose should not exceed 25-30 g, and in elderly people 15-20 g (taking into account confectionery, jams, etc.).

- With the development of side effects (nausea, flatulence, heartburn, "metallic" taste in the mouth), the intake of the sweetener should be canceled.

4.3.1.1 Sorbitol and xylitol

Sorbitol is a six-atom alcohol obtained from rowanberries, pears, apples, and plums. It is an alcohol sugar as well as xylitol. These two sweetener have approximately the same characteristics at the difference that xylitol have better effects on oral health and the prevention of several metabolic diseases

Sorbitol is a sweet, water-soluble powder made from plant extracts. It is found in small quantities in berries and fruits, most of all in mountain ash.

Participating in the metabolic processes of the body, 1 g of sorbitol forms 4 kcal of energy. Metabolized without insulin. An increase in sorbitol or xylitol intake over 30 g per day can cause a laxative effect and discomfort in the stomach. Sorbitol and xylitol can be added to hot cooked dishes. Sorbitol is inferior to sucrose in sweetness.

The inclusion of sorbitol in the sorbitol cycle can contribute to the development of cataracts, neuropathies, and microangiopathies. After 2-3 months of taking sorbitol, it is recommended to take a break of 1-2 months.

4.3.1.2 Fructose

Fructose is a sweet substance that is part of berries, fruits, and sugar. The energy value of fructose is 3.8 kcal / g. Fructose is suitable for hot cooking.

Compared to glucose, fructose is absorbed more slowly and is metabolized without insulin, therefore products containing predominantly fructose are better tolerated by patients with insulin deficiency. Fructose is a natural monosaccharide that makes up about 9% of the energy consumed by food. About 33% of edible fructose is reported to be found in fruits, vegetables, and other natural food sources.

Fructose is two times sweeter than sugar. Its daily intake should not exceed 30 g. The use of fructose more than 30 g / day leads to decompensation of diabetes mellitus with an increase in the content of total cholesterol and LDL cholesterol in the blood, an increase in the concentration of lactic acid, an accumulation of fructose and sorbitol in the lens of the eye, nerve tissue and vascular endothelium. This leads to cataracts, neuropathy, angiopathy and the accelerated development of atherosclerosis. Thus, fructose, despite its indisputable advantage over glucose and sucrose, cannot serve as a complete sweetener.

4.3.1.3 Aspartame

Aspartame is a substance consisting of two amino acids (aspartic acid and phenylalanine), which is 200 times sweeter than sugar, has no energy value and have side effects such as: neurological troubles and disturbance of protein metabolism if taken in a regular basis. One tablet of aspartame for sweetness corresponds to 3.2 g of sugar.

It is metabolized without insulin, its energy value is 3.7 kcal / g. It counteracts the development of caries. When hydrolyzed, aspartame loses its sweet taste. Hydrolysis can be prevented with organic acids and low storage temperatures. When boiling, it loses its properties. The daily dose of aspartame is 20–40 mg/kg body weight.

Some scientific reports and medical doctors reported several brain-related symptoms after an acute and/or chronic ingestion of aspartame. Aspartame is not recommended for a long-term use in diabetes patients even its advantages as a non-insulin dependent sweetener.

4.3.1.4 Saccharin

Saccharin is an imide of ortho sulfobenzoic acid. Saccharin is a crystalline powder that is 500 times sweeter than sugar, soluble in water but has a bitter taste. It does not have energy value. It is produced under various names. The daily dose of saccharin is 2.5 mg/kg body weight, that is, no more than 2 tablets. One sweetness tablet is approximately equal to one teaspoon of sugar.

Saccharin is not involved in metabolic processes. It should not be boiled due to the acquired unpleasant bitter taste. 10–20% of the saccharin taken is excreted in the feces. Saccharin accumulates in the kidneys, liver, spleen, lungs, but more in the bladder. Experimental studies indicate its carcinogenic effect on the bladder. Diseases of the liver and kidneys are contraindications to the appointment of saccharin. It is not recommended to use saccharin for children, breastfeeding and pregnant women.

4.3.1.5 Sodium cyclamate

Sodium cyclamate (daily dose of 10 mg/kg) and acesulfame (daily dose of 8 mg/kg) like saccharin are not completely absorbed by the body. They are 30-50 times sweeter than sucrose, in large doses they have a laxative effect. As sweeteners, they are rarely used at present.

4.3.1.6 Stevia extract

Natural low-calorie sugar substitute. It has a clean sweet taste, without bitterness and aftertaste. 150 times sweeter than sugar. 5 times less caloric than sugar. Stevia extract is approved for use in the manufacture of products for children from three years. Stevia extract can withstand temperatures up to 198 degrees. This is one of the main differences between sugar and artificial sweeteners (aspartame, cyclamate, saccharin, etc.), without bitterness and aftertaste.

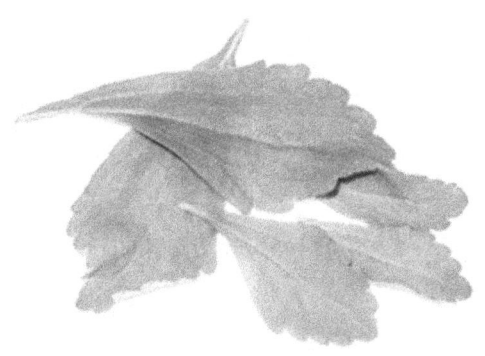

Fresh stevia leaves

Designed for use in the home kitchen when cooking, baking, as well as hot and cold drinks. Stevia extract seems to be the better solution (together with xylitol) among all the other sweeteners regarding its good value for money and the absence of side effects at least in what is currently known in the scientific literature. However, the use of sweeteners in general is not recommended regularly for long-term periods and should be used wisely, as very few data are available on sweetener currently.

4.4 Fat intake in diabetes

In the diet of patients with diabetes should be reduced intake of fat and cholesterol. In diabetes mellitus, it is undesirable to eat saturated animal fats (pork, lamb, geese, ducks) and foods rich in cholesterol (brain, liver, heart, egg yolks, etc.). The risk of developing complications of diabetes increases with LDL cholesterol levels above 115 mg / dL (3.0 mmol / L).

Fats have the highest energy value (1 g - 9 kcal) and are carriers of fat-soluble vitamins A, D, E, K. Also, they cause a feeling of fullness. In patients with diabetes, 24-30% of the energy value of the diet should be covered by fats (which is slightly lower than is usually recommended in a rational diet).

When compiling a diet, preference should be given to easily digestible fats: butter and vegetable oil. However, their amount in free form should be 30-50 g, since with food a person receives the so-called hidden fats.

Great importance is attached to the correct ratio in the diet of animal and vegetable fats. A ratio of 2/3 animal fats and 1/3 vegetable oils is desirable. In the presence of atherosclerosis, obesity, constipation, cholestatic syndrome, in older people, vegetable fats should be 1/2 of the total amount of fat.

Adequate intake of polyunsaturated fatty acids (linoleic, linolenic, arachidonic), which are indispensable nutritional factors, is necessary. These substances lower blood cholesterol and are involved in the synthesis of prostaglandins.

It is necessary to minimize the consumption of margarine.

4.5 Protein intake in diabetes

The amount of protein in the diet of patients with diabetes should be slightly higher than the physiological norm, to reduce the quota of fats and carbohydrates to ensure sufficient energy value of the diet. The recommended energy value of the diet due to proteins is 16–20% (in a rational diet - 10–15%), if the patient's renal function is normal. Proteins of animal origin should account for 55% of the total amount of proteins.

Some categories of patients require enhanced protein nutrition: children, adolescents, pregnant women, and lactating mothers, depleted, febrile, losing a lot of proteins due to some complications of diabetes (nephrotic syndrome with nephroangiopathy, malabsorption syndrome with diabetic enteropathy). In these cases, protein is introduced into the diet at the rate of 1.5–2 g / kg of the patient's body weight.

The amount of protein is limited in renal and liver failure, as well as in ketoacidosis since ketone bodies can be synthesized from some amino acids in the body. Ketogenic amino acids are leucine, isoleucine, and valine.

It should be borne in mind that glucose can form from part of the amino acids during gluconeogenesis in the patient's body.

4.6 Vitamins and minerals in diabetes

The diet of patients with diabetes should contain a sufficient amount of water- and fat-soluble vitamins. Of particular importance is vitamin B_1 (thiamine), which is actively involved in carbohydrate metabolism and the synthesis of a mediator of nerve impulses of acetylcholine. Vitamin B_1 is found in the greatest quantities in yeast, wholemeal bread, bran, and beans.

It is necessary that a sufficient amount of micronutrients arrives with food, among which zinc, copper, and manganese are important since they indirectly lower blood sugar. Zinc is part of insulin, increases the immunobiological reactivity of the body and has a lipotropic effect. Zinc is rich in yeast, eggs, cereals, legumes, mushrooms, and Dutch cheese. Manganese enhances the hypoglycemic effect of insulin, stimulates oxidative processes in the body, increases its reactivity, and has lipotropic and hypocholesterolemic effects. Manganese is found in cereals, cereals, raspberries, black currants. Copper also enhances the oxidative processes in the body and increases its reactivity, improves the antitoxic function of the liver, participates in the synthesis of hemoglobin, and inhibits insulinase that destroys insulin. Food sources of copper are nuts,

The content of sodium chloride in the diet of patients with diabetes according to WHO is only 6 g / day. However, domestic diets allow the consumption of salt up to 10-12 g / day.

4.7 Fluid intake in diabetes

The recommended amount of free fluid is about 1.5 l / day. They limit fluid only with edema and impaired renal function.

The danger of excessive intake of alcoholic beverages by patients with diabetes should be emphasized. Alcohol intoxication can lead to severe hypoglycemia, even in healthy people.

There are several causes of alcohol hypoglycemia.

- Alcohol stimulates insulin secretion.

- In chronic alcoholism and diabetes, depletion of glycogen stores in the liver is often observed.

- Alcohol blocks the stage of gluconeogenesis, in which alanine and lactic acid are converted into pyruvic acid, and prevents glycerol from being included in gluconeogenesis. In this case, lactic acidosis can develop.

- Ethanol can contribute to the development or deepening of ketoacidosis.

For these reasons, alcohol is strictly forbidden to patients receiving biguanides, which in themselves can cause lactic acidosis. Drinking alcohol while using sulfonamides can also be harmful. On the one hand, ethanol potentiates the sugar-lowering effect of sulfonylurea, and on the other hand, these drugs reduce alcohol tolerance. One of the sulfa drugs - chlorpropamide after drinking alcohol can cause severe facial flushing, a rush of blood to the head, suffocation, and a decrease in blood pressure.

4.8 Energy value of the diet in diabetes patient

The energy value of the diet of a patient with diabetes should correspond to the physiological energy needs of a healthy person of the appropriate gender, age, and profession.

Tab.1: Calculation of energy expenditure for a patient with diabetes in kcal.

Fatness	Number of Kcal according to the activity level		
	Inactivity	Moderate activity	Significant activity
Excess	20–25	30	35
Normal	30	35	40
Lowered	35	40	45-50

DIET THERAPY FOR DIABETES

With diabetes, diet and the correct distribution of the energy value of the diet during the day are of great importance. Fractional nutrition avoids large simultaneous loads on the insular apparatus of the pancreas.

With 6 meals a day, the following scheme is recommended: first breakfast - 25% of the daily energy intensity of the diet; second breakfast - 10-15%; lunch - 25%; afternoon tea - 5-10%; dinner - 25%; second dinner - 5-10%. If the patient, due to circumstances, is forced to consume the bulk of food at breakfast or late lunch (upon returning from work), then the energy value of the diet can be distributed as follows: breakfast - 30%; second breakfast - 10-15%; afternoon tea - 10-15%; dinner (late lunch) - 30%; second dinner - 10-15%.

5.1 General dietary requirements for diabetes

- Frequent meals - 4-5 times a day at the same time.

- Individual distribution of carbohydrates during the day.

- Controlled caloric intake of the daily diet, the optimal ratio of protein, fat, and carbohydrates in the diet. If necessary, calorie restriction up to 1800-2000 calories.

- Exclusion of rapidly absorbed carbohydrates (sugar, sweets, confectionery), limiting the total number of carbohydrates.

- An increase in the total amount of protein in the diet, a controlled ratio of animal to vegetable protein.

- Limitation of fat in the diet, the predominant use of low fat and nonfat products.

- Enrichment of the diet with vitamins and minerals due to the inclusion of seafood, raw vegetables, fruits, berries, broths of wild rose, black currant.

- An increase in dietary fiber (up to 40-50 g per day) due to the widespread inclusion of vegetables, as well as wheat bran.

5.2 Diet Therapy Tactics for Diabetes

In the absence of contraindications, the patient with diabetes is prescribed a diabetes diet

The trial diet contains too many fats, but a dramatically reduced amount of carbohydrates, which reduces the load on the insular apparatus of the pancreas. Against the background of a trial diet, fasting blood sugar and daily urine for sugar are examined at least 1 time in 5 days.

With normalization of carbohydrate metabolism, this diet is treated for 2-3 weeks, after which it is gradually expanded, adding 1 XE every 3-7 days (depending on body weight). Before each new increase, blood and urine for sugar are examined. Having expanded the trial diet by 12 XEs, stand for 2 months, then add another 4 XEs with an interval of 3-7 days. Further expansion of the diet, if necessary, is carried out after 1 year.

When treated in hospitals, patients with diabetes should receive the basic version of a standard diet. For patients with type II diabetes mellitus and obesity, a low-calorie diet option is recommended (up to 1800-2000 calories).

All variants of diets with reduced energy value have disadvantages, so it is important to be able to individually calculate the diet for a particular patient with diabetes, who is overweight. To do this, it is necessary to determine the physiological need for energy, reduce it by 30% and calculate the chemical composition of the diet. With the lack of effectiveness of such a diet, the energy value can be reduced by 40 or 50% of the physiological norm.

In order to more quickly reduce excess weight, it is recommended to include fasting days in the course of diet therapy: meat, fish, cottage cheese, kefir. It is recommended to spend fasting days once a week, while it is better to observe an active motor regime. The process of weight loss at home should take place under the supervision of a doctor and not exceed a loss of 2-3 kg of weight per month.

Fasting days can be carried out in the presence of obesity and for patients receiving insulin. On unloading days, the dose of insulin administered must be reduced. The amount of insulin administered on the day of discharge must be determined by the doctor.

5.3 Features of diet therapy for patients receiving insulin

Particular attention should be paid to diet therapy in patients receiving insulin.

On an outpatient basis, patients receiving insulin of short and medium duration of action must strictly observe two rules:

1. The amount of foods rich in carbohydrates should be constant every day. To diversify the carbohydrate part of the diet, you can use the table of interchangeability of products for carbohydrates.

2. These products must be properly distributed throughout the day by the curve of action of the insulin used.

Failure to comply with the rules can lead to hypo- or hyperglycemia.

For patients receiving insulin, an insulin diet is recommended. This diet is excessive in calories for almost all women, as well as for men engaged in mental work. This once again proves the need to individualize the nutrition of patients. For the insulin diet, the same foods and dishes are allowed as for diabetes diet. Instead of sugar, various sweeteners are used, but each patient receiving insulin should have sugar for stopping possible hypoglycemia.

Currently, in hospitals, patients with diabetes mellitus are advised to use a variant of a diet with a high protein content (high-protein diet) when treating insulin. However, it should be remembered that not all patients treated with insulin have an increased protein requirement. Such a diet is more suitable for patients with infectious complications and diabetic nephropathy with nephrotic syndrome.

5.3.1 Diet for patients receiving insulin of various durations of action

5.3.1.1 When taking simple insulin

- 8.00 - protein breakfast (egg, cottage cheese, meat), insulin injection.
- 9.00 - carbohydrates (porridge or potatoes).
- 11.30 - carbohydrates (bread).
- 14.00 - lunch without bread.
- 17.00 - injection of insulin.
- 18.00 - carbohydrates (porridge or potatoes).
- 20.30 - carbohydrates (bread).

5.3.1.2 When taking insulin for up to 24 hours

- 8.00 - insulin injection.
- 9.00 - carbohydrates.

- 11.30 - carbohydrates.

- 14.00 - carbohydrates.

- 18.00 - carbohydrates.

- 22.30–23.00 - carbohydrates at bedtime (usually bread) for the prevention of night hypoglycemia.

5.3.1.3 When taking insulin with a duration of action of 30–36 hours

- 7.00 carbohydrates immediately after rising to the introduction of insulin to avoid morning hypoglycemia.

- 8.00 insulin injection.

- 9.00 carbohydrates.

- 11.30 carbohydrates.

- 14.00 carbohydrates.

- 18.00 carbohydrates.

- 22.30-23.00 carbohydrates at bedtime (usually bread) for the prevention of nocturnal hypoglycemia.

5.4 Diet therapy for patients with a threat of diabetic coma

If there is a threat of a diabetic coma, the amount of fat in the diet is limited to 30 g, and protein to 50 g, since ketone bodies can be synthesized from fats and ketogenic amino acids in the body. The amount of carbohydrates, in this case, is 300 g, mainly due to easily digestible. During this period, the patient is allowed foods and dishes that were forbidden in everyday nutrition (sugar, jam, semolina and, rice porridge, etc.) due to the antiketogenic effect of carbohydrates.

In pre coma, only carbohydrate foods are recommended, fats and proteins are completely excluded.

On the first day after the elimination of the diabetic coma and the use of rehydration, detoxification and hypoglycemic therapy, alkaline mineral waters, potassium-rich vegetable and fruit juices, fruit drinks, jelly are shown.

From the second day they give vegetables and fruits in mashed form (potato, carrot, applesauce), crackers, mashed soups, semolina, rice and oatmeal, kefir.

From the 5th day, protein dishes are included in the diet: cottage cheese, boiled fish, protein omelet, chopped meat, and chicken.

Not earlier than the 10th day free fats (butter and vegetable oil) are introduced into the diet.

5.5 Diet therapy for possible hypoglycemia

In the presence of precursors of hypoglycemia (feelings of hunger, weakness, fever, sweating), you can limit yourself to one or two pieces of bread or rolls (25-50 g). After taking bread or rolls, the manifestations of hypoglycemia should be eliminated after 10-15 minutes.

With more pronounced manifestations of hypoglycemia (headache and dizziness, severe pallor, paresthesia, muscle tremors), it is necessary to give sweet warm tea (2-3 teaspoons of sugar per cup of tea). After taking sweet tea, improvement occurs in 5-7 minutes.

If the patient is close to loss of consciousness, it is necessary to immediately appoint 100% sugar syrup (2-3 tsp.). The use of sugar syrup improves the patient's condition in a few minutes.

With the development of hypoglycemic shock or coma, the effect can be obtained only from jet intravenous administration of a concentrated (20-40%) glucose solution. With intravenous administration of glucose, the patient regains consciousness "on the tip of the needle", i.e. directly during the injection.

5.6 Diabetes Prevention

Lifestyle changes in high-risk patients can prevent the development of type II diabetes mellitus by more than 2 times.

Prevention of diabetes involves the following areas:

- Weight loss of 5% or more in obese patients.
- Decrease in fat intake up to 30% or less of the daily calorie intake.
- Reducing saturated fat intake to 10% or less of daily calories.
- Increase in dietary fiber intake.

- Conducting physical exercises of medium intensity up to 30 minutes or more per day.

- Correction of existing dyslipidemia.

- Hypertension control.

- Compliance with the regime of work and rest.

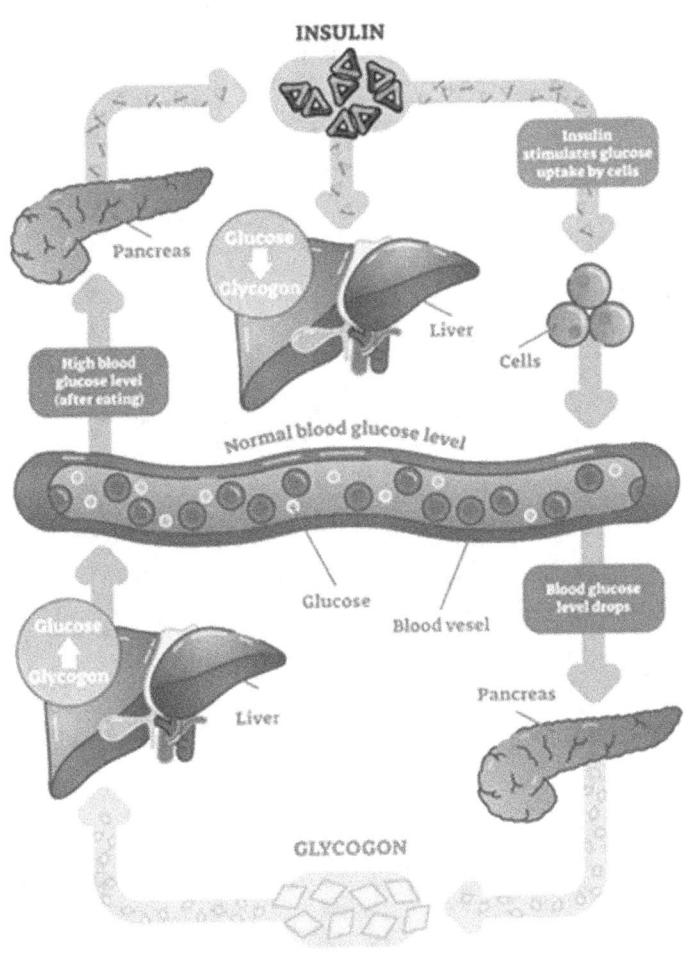

PHYTOTHERAPY FOR DIABETES

For the prevention and treatment of diabetes for many years, teas from the following berries and plants have been recommended: wild strawberries, dioica nettle, burdock, oats, dandelion, plantain, yarrow, beans, chicory, blueberries, and rose hips.

It is recommended to include salads from leaves of dandelion, nettle, chicory, wild highlander, and medicago officinalis in the diet. These plants are rich in tocopherol, ascorbic acid, compounds of phosphorus, iron, calcium, aluminum, manganese, organic compounds (inulin, magnesium, inositol, flavoxanthin, wax, etc.).

6.1 Recommendations for the use of medicinal plants for diabetes

- Ginseng (pharmacy tincture) - 15-20 drops in the morning and afternoon. Extract (pharmacy) - 5-10 drops in the morning and afternoon.

- Eleutherococcus (extract) - 1 / 4-1 / 2 tsp. morning and afternoon.

- Golden root (Rhodiola Rosea) (pharmacy extract) - 1/4-1/2 tsp. at the reception in the morning and afternoon.

- Stinging nettle (7 g of dry chopped herbs in a glass of boiling water, steam for 15-20 minutes, drink 1 tbsp. 3 times a day).

- Dandelion (roots, grass). 6 g of dry crushed raw materials per glass of water, boil for 10 minutes, insist for 30 minutes, take 1 tbsp. 1 4 times a day before meals.

- Chicory (grass - as food in the form of salads, and roots (dried and ground) - as a substitute for coffee).

- As hypoglycemic agents, it is recommended to use leaves of Manchurian and Walnut, lingonberry, blueberry, blueberry, St. John's wort, elecampane, wild strawberry, bean pods, burdock, and lure.

- The herbal remedies for diabetes include the fruits, seeds, and berries of black elderberry, blueberry, wild strawberry, gooseberry, hemp, mountain ash, mulberry, raspberry, blackberry, citrus, lentil, celery roots, barley extract, cabbage, chestnut, alfalfa, oats, spinach, and others

- A positive effect is noted when using tea of the following composition: blueberry leaves - 4 parts, bean pods - 4 parts, ordinary strawberry leaves - 3 parts, yarrow grass - 1 part, burdock root - 3 parts, dioecious nettle leaves - 4 parts, root common dandelion - 2 parts, flowering oat panicle - 4 parts, bony leaves - 4 parts, rose hips - 4 parts.

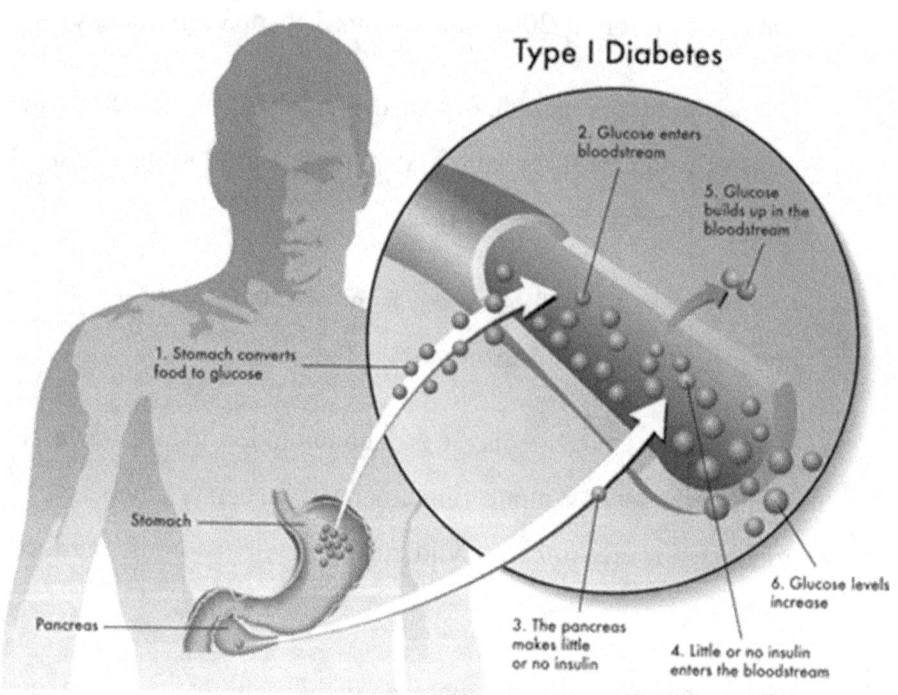

TYPE OF DIET USED FOR THE TREATMENT OF DIABETES

7.1 Diabetes Diet

7.1.1 Indications

This diet is used in the treatment of diseases such as type 2 diabetes mellitus of mild to moderate severity, joint diseases, a large group of allergic diseases (bronchial asthma, etc.).

7.1.2 Purpose

Creating conditions conducive to the normalization of carbohydrate metabolism, determining the patient's tolerance to carbohydrates.

7.1.3 General characteristic

A diet with energy moderately reduced due to easily digestible carbohydrates and animal fats, except sugar and sweets, and the use of xylitol. With the physiological norm of vitamins and minerals. Sugar, jam, confectionery, and other products containing a lot of sugar are excluded.

Sugar is replaced with sugar substitutes: xylitol, stevia extract and in a lesser extent fructose.

The culinary processing is diverse: cooking, stewing, baking and roasting without breading.

Eating 5-6 times a day.

With diabetes in obese patients, therapeutic nutrition coincides with the treatment of obese patients.

7.1.4 Chemical composition and energy value

Proteins 100 g, fats 70-80 g (of which 25 g vegetable), carbohydrates 300 g mainly due to complex, simple carbohydrates are excluded or sharply limited; calorie content 2300 kcal; retinol 0.3 mg, carotene 12 mg, thiamine 1.5 mg, riboflavin 2.1 mg, nicotinic acid 18 mg, ascorbic acid 100 mg; sodium 3.7 g, potassium 4 g, calcium 0.8 g, phosphorus 1.3 g, iron 15 mg. Free fluid 1.5 liters.

7.1.5 Recommended foods

- Bread and bread from the product - mainly from whole grains or with the addition of bran; Diabetic varieties of bread: protein-bran, protein-wheat.

- Soups - mainly vegetarian or on bone broth from prefabricated vegetables, borscht, pickles, okroshka, bean (once or twice a week on meat or fish broth).

- Dishes from meat and poultry - low-fat varieties of meat and poultry - beef, lamb, pork, chicken, turkey, boiled, seasoned, baked rabbit (fried once a week). Goose, duck, animal internal organs, brains are not recommended.

- Sausages - low in fat.

- Dishes from fish - a variety of sea and river fish - cod, saffron cod, ice, pikeperch, pike mainly in boiled, aspic, baked form.

- Vegetables, greens - cauliflower and white cabbage, leafy lettuce, eggplant, zucchini, watermelon, pumpkin, cucumbers, tomatoes, green peas, beans, beans, lentils, bell peppers, onions, beets, carrots, parsley, dill, celery, estragon, cilantro. Limited to potatoes.

- Dishes from berries and fruits - unsweetened varieties of berries and fruits: apples, pears, quinces, oranges, lemons, grapefruit, pomegranate, cherry, plum, peaches, currants, lingonberries, raspberries, strawberries, cranberries, raw rowan, dried, in in the form of compotes, jelly, jelly without added sugar, using sweeteners. Bananas, figs are not recommended, grapes, raisins are limited.

- Dishes from cereals, pasta - oat, buckwheat, "Hercules", millet, diet pasta with bran, in the form of a variety of cereals, casseroles, taking into account the total amount of carbohydrates in the diet.

- Dishes from eggs - one egg per day, soft-boiled or as an omelet, scrambled eggs, to be added to dishes.

- Dairy products - mostly low-fat or low-fat - fresh cottage cheese or in the form of cheesecakes, puddings, cottage cheese (without added sugar), kefir, yogurt, milk, cheese, cream, low-fat butter.

- Confectionery - only dietary with sugar substitutes (biscuits, cookies, xylitol wafers, marmalade, sweets with sugar substitutes).

- Fats - butter (peasant), sandwich margarine, sunflower, corn, olive oil in its natural form.

- Drinks - tea, tea with milk, coffee drink, tomato juice, fruit and berry juices without sugar, rosehip broth, soft drinks without sugar, mineral water.

- Snacks - salads, vinaigrettes, jellied low-fat fish and meat, soaked herring, cheese, low-fat sausage, vegetable caviar.

7.1.6 Excluded foods

- Sugar, sweets, chocolate, confectionery with added sugar, muffin, pies, jam, ice cream, and other sweets.

- Butter dough products.

- Goose, duck, smoked meat, salted fish.

- Baked milk, cream, fermented baked milk, sweet yogurt, ayran.

- Meat and cooking fats.

- Strong and greasy broths.
- Milk cheeses, cream, sweet curd cheeses.
- Fatty meats, fish, poultry, sausages, salted fish.
- Rice, semolina, pasta.
- Salted and pickled vegetables. Pickled and sauerkraut.
- Spicy, spicy, smoked snacks, mustard, pepper.
- Grapes, raisins, figs, bananas and other sweet fruits.
- Juices and fruit water with added sugar.
- Alcoholic drinks.

7.1.7 Approximate one-day diet for patients with diabetes

- Breakfast: buckwheat porridge (cereal - 40 g, butter - 10 g), meat (or fish) paste (meat - 60 g, butter - 5 g), tea with milk (milk - 50 g).
- 11 hours: a glass of kefir.
- Lunch: vegetable soup (vegetable oil - 5 g, soaked potatoes - 50 g, cabbage - 100 g, carrots - 25 g, sour cream - 5 g, tomato - 20 g), boiled meat - 100 g, soaked potatoes - 150 g, oil - 5 g, apple - 200 g.
- 17 h: yeast drink.

- Dinner: zrazy from carrots with cottage cheese (carrots - 75 g, cottage cheese - 50 g, semolina - 8 g, rye crackers - 5 g, egg - 1 piece). Boiled fish - 100 g, cabbage - 150 g, vegetable oil - 10 g, tea with xylitol.

- At night: a glass of kefir.

- Bread per day - 250 g (mainly rye).

7.1.8 Approximate set of products per day for patients with diabetes

- Butter 20 g

- Milk 200 ml.

- Kefir 200 ml.

- Curd 100 g.

- Sour cream 40 g

- Groats 50 g.

- Potato 200 g

- Tomatoes 20 g.

- Cabbage 600 g

- Carrots 75 g.

- Greens 25 g.

- Beef 150 g.

- Fish 100 g

- White bread 100 g.

- Black bread 200 g

7.2 Trial diet

7.2.1 Chemical composition and value

Proteins - 116 g; carbohydrates - 130, fats - 136 g, energy value - 2170–2208 kcal. The ratio of proteins / fats / carbohydrates = 1: 1.3: 1.2.

Against the background of a trial diet, fasting blood sugar and daily urine for sugar are examined at least 1 time in 5 days.

With normalization of carbohydrate metabolism, this diet is treated for 2-3 weeks, after which it is gradually expanded, adding 1 XE every 3-7 days (depending on body weight). Before each new increase, blood and urine for sugar are examined. Having expanded the trial diet by 12 XEs, stand for 2 months, then add another 4 XEs with an interval of 3-7 days. Further expansion of the diet, if necessary, is carried out after 1 year.

7.2.2 Daily set of products of the trial diet

- Meat, fish 250 g.

- Curd 300 g

- Cheese 25 g.
- Milk, kefir 500 ml.
- Butter and vegetable oil 60 g.
- Vegetables (except potatoes and legumes) 800 g.
- Fruits (except grapes, bananas, persimmons, figs) 300 g.
- Black bread 100 g.

7.3 Insulin diet

7.3.1 Indications for the Insulin diet

Recommended for patients with insulin-dependent diabetes mellitus receiving large doses of insulin.

7.3.2 Chemical composition and energy value of insulin diet

The diet is close in chemical composition to a rational table.

Proteins - 100 g, fats - 80–100 g, carbohydrates - 400–450 g, energy value 2700–3100 kcal.

On the insulin diet, the same foods and dishes are allowed as on the diabetes diet.

Instead of sugar, various sugar substitutes are used, but each patient receiving insulin should have sugar to stop possible hypoglycemia.

The majority of carbohydrates must be given with the first breakfast and lunch. Before these meals, insulin is prescribed. With the introduction of insulin before dinner, you should leave food at night to prevent possible hypoglycemic reactions.

If there is a risk of developing a diabetic coma, the amount of fat in the diet should be reduced to 30 g, protein to 50 g. The carbohydrate content should not exceed 300 g. At the same time, the dose of insulin administered is increased.

7.4 Option Diabetes Diet for patients with bronchial asthma

7.4.1 Chemical composition and energy value

The calorie content of food is calculated by physiological norms of the need for sources of energy substances, but with the restriction of sugar and its products and dishes. The average calorie table of patients with bronchial asthma is 2600-2700 kcal. They should be represented by proteins in an amount of 100-130 g, fats - 85 g, carbohydrates - 300 g. The amount of sodium chloride is 10-11 g. The liquid must be consumed up to 1.5-1.8 l.

The total daily amount of food should be divided into 4-5 receptions.

7.4.2 Recommended products and dishes

- First courses - any soups and other dishes prepared based on broths from lean types of meat and poultry should contain a minimum amount of extractives.

- Second courses are prepared from meat, fish, and poultry of low-fat varieties.

- Chicken meat and chicken egg protein are often food allergens, but if their etiological role in the origin of asthma is not identified, their use is allowed, but it is necessary to limit their amount in the patient's diet.

- Milk and dairy products are used with caution, given that milk protein is an allergen and can be dangerous for people with an allergic predisposition. Goat, mare's milk should also be used with caution.

- Side dishes for the second dish can be prepared from vegetables, but in this case, one should be guided by the need to prefer fried boiling, stewing, steaming.

7.4.3 Excluded foods and meals for patients with bronchial asthma

- You should limit the use of free carbohydrates - sugar, honey, sweets (ice cream), fried foods and smoked foods.

- If possible, limit the use of flour products - buns, pies, cookies, cakes and similar products and dishes.

- Lamb, fatty pork broths, soups seasoned with cereals and noodles are excluded.

- It is preferable to refuse such cooking methods as roasting, eating very spicy, salty foods, using spices and seasonings, hot sauces, eating canned food (stewed meat, canned fish and similar foods).

- If the etiological role of milk as a food allergen is reliably known, it is, if possible, excluded from consumption (both directly and as part of various dishes).

- Often the use of alcoholic beverages (even in small quantities) is a factor that provokes the development of a typical asthma attack, so people suffering from bronchial asthma should completely exclude the intake of alcoholic beverages, even low-alcohol ones (beer).

- Among the appetizers, salted fish, pickled mushrooms, vegetables, spicy types of vegetables and other appetizers are excluded.

- Hot peppers, mustard, spices are completely excluded from the diet.

- Of fruits, the use of grapes, citrus fruits (oranges, lemons, grapefruits, juices, jams and other products made from them) is limited, strawberries, raspberries, dates, raisins, bananas.

- Limit the use of honey, jam, jam, confiture, chocolate, cocoa.

- Among drinks, juices from forbidden fruits or berries, cocoa, coffee, hot chocolate are limited.

7.4.4 Approximate one-day diet for patients with asthma

7.4.4.1 Option 1

- First breakfast: semolina porridge - 150 g, butter - 20 g, low-fat cottage cheese - 100 g, tea with lemon - 180 ml.

- Second breakfast: pumpkin casserole with apples - 100 g, boiled meat paste - 80 g.

- Lunch: vegetable okroshka - 180 g, stuffed cabbage stuffed with boiled meat - 200 g, vegetable stew - 100 g, jelly from applesauce - 180 ml.

- Snack: vinaigrette with vegetable oil - 100 g.

- Dinner: boiled potatoes - 200 g, mushrooms in sour cream - 150 g, apple juice - 180 ml.

- At night: kefir - 180 ml.

7.4.4.2 Option 2

- First breakfast: rice porridge - 150 g with butter - 20 g, tea with lemon - 180 ml.

- Second breakfast: pilaf with fruits - 100 g, baked apples - 75 g.

- Lunch: vegetarian borsch - 180 ml, sour cream - 10 g, zucchini stuffed with boiled meat - 200 g, baked carrot cutlets - 100 g, dried fruit jelly - 180 ml.

- Afternoon snack: blackcurrant jelly - 180 g.

- Dinner: boiled potatoes - 200 g, goulash from boiled meat - 150 g, compote from fresh apples - 180 ml.

- At night: kefir - 150 ml.

7.4.4.3 Option 3

- First breakfast: semolina porridge - 150 g with butter - 20 g, rosehip broth - 180 ml.

- Second breakfast: potato casserole with cottage cheese - 100 g, boiled tongue - 40 g.

- Lunch: green cabbage soup - 180 ml, pancakes with boiled meat - 150 g, liver pudding with carrots - 50 g, dried fruit jelly - 180 g.

- Snack: baked carrot cutlets - 100 g.

- Dinner: boiled potatoes - 200 g, meatballs stewed in sauce - 150 g, fresh apple compote - 180 ml.

- At night: kefir - 150ml.

7.4.5 Recipes for dietary dishes

7.4.5.1 First meal

- **The broth is transparent.**

    Required: 1 kg of beef with bones, 200 g of beef (pulp), 1 egg white, 1 carrot, 1/2 bunch of parsley, 1/2 bunch of celery, 1 onion, 4 peas of allspice, 1 bay leaf, 3 l of water, salt.

    Cooking: Put washed and chopped bones, meat in a saucepan, pour water and boil. Then drain the broth and again pour the meat with hot boiled water. When the water boils, remove the foam, add salt and cook over low heat for at least 3 hours. Put chopped greens in the middle of cooking. At the end of cooking, put pepper, bay leaf. When the broth is boiled, remove the pan from the fire, remove the bones and meat, let the broth stand. Then strain through a metal frequent sieve. If the cooked broth is not transparent enough, it can be clarified with egg white. Use this broth as a base for making soups. For the broth, you can use veal, lean beef.

- **The pickle is dietary.**

    Required: 200 g of weak broth, 20 g of onion, 10 g of oil, 20 g of carrots, 20 g of herbs to taste, 50 g of pickles, 50 g of potatoes, 20 g of pearl barley, 30 g of sour cream.

    Cooking: Cut carrots and onions into small slices and simmer lightly. Peel the cucumbers, cut into thin slices and, after pouring a little broth, cook for 10-15 minutes. In the rest of the broth, boil the cereal with potatoes and put the cucumbers and carrots with herbs there. Let the soup boil and season with sour cream.

- **Summer diet soup.**

  Required: 300 g of broth, 15 g of oil, 20 g of onion, 40 g of carrots, 120 g of cabbage, 60 g of potatoes, 40 g of tomatoes, 30 g of sour cream, parsley.

  Cooking: Stew finely chopped onions in a small amount of oil with added water. Then add sliced carrots and stew until half cooked. Cut cabbage and potatoes into small cubes and put in boiling broth, put the stewed vegetables there and cook until cooked. When serving, put sour cream and finely chopped parsley in the soup.

- **Cabbage soup mashed.**

  Required: 200 g of weak broth, 10 g of oil, 20 g of carrots, 10 g of tomato puree, 50 g of beets, 20 g of onions, 60 g of cabbage, 60 g of potatoes, 3 g of flour, 30 g of sour cream, bay leaf.

  Cooking: Sliced carrots and beets in a pan, add oil, tomato puree, salt, and stew, closing the lid until the vegetables are soft. Fry onion in oil and mix with stewed vegetables. Then pour the broth and add finely chopped cabbage and potatoes, put a bay leaf. Boil cabbage soup until vegetables are ready. Then rub the cabbage soup through a sieve, season with toasted flour, salt to taste and bring to a boil again. When serving, add sour cream to cabbage soup.

- **Soup with meatballs.**

Required: 300 g of broth, 10 g of oil, 70 g of low-fat beef or veal, 200 g of potatoes, 1/2 eggs, 20 g of onions, parsley.

Cooking: Skip the meat through a meat grinder, add half of the finely chopped onion, egg, salt and mix thoroughly. Roll small meatballs from minced meat and cook them in the broth. Boil the rest of the broth, put the potatoes in it and the remaining onion, which was previously sautéed in oil. When the soup is cooked, put meatballs in it and sprinkle with finely chopped parsley.

- **Fish soup with mashed meatballs.**

Required: 250 g of fish broth, 20 g of onion, 100 g of fish, 10 g of bread, 20 g of milk, 5 g of egg white, 200 g of potatoes, 30 g of sour cream, 5 g of oil, herbs.

Cooking: Fry the onion in oil, put in fish stock, add chopped potatoes and cook. Pass the fish through a meat grinder along with a roll soaked in milk, add the egg, salt and mix the minced fish well. Make meatballs and cook them separately in the broth. Then put the meatballs in the soup and add sour cream. Serving to the table, sprinkle with herbs.

- **Vegetable soup with rice broth.**

Required: 150 g of potatoes, 70 g of carrots, 30 g of rice, 1 glass of milk, 1 tbsp. l oil, 1/2 egg yolk.

Cooking: Rinse and boil rice until cooked. Then wipe, mix with boiled and grated potatoes and carrots, dilute with boiling milk, season with yolk and butter. Giving to the table, garnish with chopped greens.

7.4.5.2 Second meal

- **Veal cutlets steam.**

Required: 200 g of veal, 20 g of bread, 30 g of milk, 5 g of butter.

Cooking: Rinse the meat, cut into small pieces and pass through a meat grinder. Add the loaf soaked in milk and once again mince the minced meat through a meat grinder. Pour in the rest of the milk and melted butter, add salt and mix. Make cutlets and lay them on the wire rack of the double boiler. Put a double boiler on fire and cook cutlets for at least 15 minutes. Serve the patties with butter.

- **Steam meatballs.**

Required: 200 g lean beef, 30 g rice, 20 g butter.

Cooking: Pass the meat through a meat grinder, boil the rice in water until tender, then drain and mix with the meat, again pass through the meat grinder, add a little water to the minced meat and add salt. Mix the mass well and make a few bollards. Steam meatballs. When serving, pour sour cream.

- **Chicken Steam Chops.**

Required: 300 g of chicken meat, 20 g of stale rolls, 20 g of milk, 15 g of butter.

Cooking: Pass the chicken meat through a meat grinder, add the loaf soaked in milk, skip again and put a little butter, mix well and form the meatballs. Steam. Serve the meatballs with a vegetable side dish.

- **Fish baked in the oven.**

Requires: 1 kg of sturgeon or pike perch, 2 tbsp. l sour cream, 1 tbsp. l oils, salt, parsley.

Cooking: Put the cleaned fish skin down on a greased baking sheet. Grease with sour cream on top, salt and pour with melted butter. Put in the oven and bake for at least 30 minutes. Before serving, cut into pieces and garnish with parsley.

- **Boiled meat baked in sauce.**

Required: 150 grams of lean beef, 70 grams of milk, 5 grams of flour, 100 grams of apples, 1 tbsp. l butter.

Cooking: Boil the meat and cut into small slices, then prepare the sauce from milk and flour. Peel the apples from the skin and core and cut into thin circles. After this, grease the pan with butter, put apple circles on the bottom, put meat mixed with apples on apples. Top with sauce and bake.

- **Diet pudding.**

Required: 130 g of zucchini, 70 g of apples, 30 g of milk, 1 tbsp. l butter, 15 g semolina, 1/2 egg, 40 g sour cream.

Cooking: Zucchini peel, chop and stew with milk until half ready. Then add chopped apples and simmer for another 3-4 minutes, then pour semolina and hold the pan under the lid on the edge of the stove for 5 minutes, then cool. Add the yolk and whipped protein separately, mix the mass, put in a mold greased with oil, and bake. Serve with sour cream to the table.

- **Potato zrazy "Surprise".**

  Required: 100 g of veal, 250 g of potatoes, greens.

  Cooking: Boil the meat and mince it. Boil the potatoes, wipe and add chopped greens. Form the prepared potato mass in circles and put the minced meat in the middle. Put in a steam bath and bake.

- **Dumplings are lazy.**

  Required: 100 g of cottage cheese, 10 g of wheat flour, 2 g of sour cream, 10 g of sugar, 1 egg.

  Cooking: Grind the cottage cheese, mix with the egg and add flour and sugar. Form a roller from this mass and cut it into small pieces. Put the dumplings in boiling water and bring to a boil. As soon as the dumplings come up, take them out and serve with sour cream.

7.4.5.3 Dessert

Kissel berry.

Required: 50 g of fresh berries, 15 g of sugar, 6 g of potato starch.

Cooking: Rub the berries and strain the juice through cheesecloth. Boil the extracts in water, strain and boil jelly from the broth. When the jelly has cooled, pour in the berry juice.

7.5 High Protein Diet

7.5.1 High Protein Diet Indications

- Condition after gastrectomy for peptic ulcer in 2–4 months in the presence of dumping syndrome, cholecystitis, hepatitis.
- Chronic enteritis in the presence of a pronounced violation of the functional state of the digestive system.
- Celiac enteropathy.
- Chronic pancreatitis in remission.
- Chronic glomerulonephritis of the nephrotic type in the stage of decaying exacerbation without the impaired nitrogen excretory function of the kidneys.
- Type 1 and type 2 diabetes without concomitant obesity and impaired renal excretory function.
- Rheumatism with a low degree of activity of the process with a prolonged course of the disease without impaired circulation.
- Rheumatism in the stage of fading exacerbation.
- Pulmonary tuberculosis.
- Suppurative processes.
- Anemia of various etiologies.
- Burn disease.

7.5.2 High Protein Diet Overview

A diet with high protein content, a normal amount of fat, complex carbohydrates and a restriction of easily digestible carbohydrates. Refined carbohydrates (sugar) are excluded.

Limit table salt (6-8 g / day), chemical and mechanical irritants of the stomach and biliary tract. Dishes are cooked boiled, stewed, baked, steamed, mashed and non-mashed. The temperature of hot dishes is not more than 60–65 ° C, cold dishes - not lower than 15 ° C.

Free liquid - 1.5–2 liters.

Diet - 4-6 times a day.

7.5.3 Chemical composition and energy value

Proteins - 110–120 g (animals - 45–50 g), fats 80–90 g (vegetable - 30 g), carbohydrates - 250–330 g (simple - 30–40 g), energy value - 2080–2690 kcal.

7.6 Main option for a standard diet

7.6.1 Indications for the main option of the standard diet

- Chronic gastritis, peptic ulcer of the stomach and duodenum in remission.
- Chronic intestinal diseases with a predominance of IBS with predominant constipation.
- Acute cholecystitis and hepatitis are recovering.
- Chronic hepatitis with mild signs of liver failure.

- Chronic cholecystitis, cholelithiasis.

- Gout, uric acid diathesis, nephrolithiasis, hyperuricemia, phosphaturia.

- Type II diabetes mellitus without concomitant overweight or obesity.

- Diseases of the cardiovascular system with mild circulatory disorders.

- Hypertonic disease.

- IHD, atherosclerosis of the coronary arteries of the heart, brain, peripheral vessels.

- Acute infectious diseases. Febrile conditions.

7.6.2 General characteristics of the main version of the standard diet

A diet with a physiological content of proteins, fats, and carbohydrates, enriched with vitamins, minerals, vegetable fiber (vegetables, fruits).

When prescribing a diet for patients with diabetes mellitus, refined carbohydrates (sugar) are excluded.

In the diet, nitrogenous extractives, table salt (6–8 g / day), foods rich in essential oils are limited, spicy seasonings, spinach, sorrel, and smoked foods are excluded.

Dishes are cooked in boiled form or steamed, baked. The temperature of hot dishes is not more than 60–65 ° C, cold dishes - not lower than 15 ° C.

Free liquid - 1.5–2 liters.

The rhythm of nutrition is fractional, 4-6 times a day.

7.6.3 Chemical composition and energy value

Protein - 85–90 g (animals 40–45 g); carbohydrates 300–350 (mono- and disaccharides 50–60 g) fats 85–90 g (vegetable - 40–45 g, energy consumption 2170–2480 kcal.

7.7 Low-calorie standard diet option (low-calorie diet)

7.7.1 Indications for a low-calorie diet

- Various degrees of alimentary obesity in the absence of pronounced complications from the digestive system, blood circulation and other diseases that require the appointment of special nutritional regimes.

- Type 2 diabetes with obesity.

- Cardiovascular disease in the presence of overweight.

7.7.2 General characteristic of a low-calorie diet

A diet with a moderate limitation of energy value (1300-1600 kcal) mainly due to fats and carbohydrates.

Simple sugars are excluded, animal fats, table salt are limited (3-5 g / day). Vegetable fats, dietary fiber (raw vegetables, fruits, food bran) are included. Food is cooked boiled or steamed, without salt.

Free fluid is limited to 0.8–1.5 l / day.

Diet 4-6 times a day.

7.7.3 Chemical composition and energy value

Proteins: 70–80 g (including animals 40 g). Fats: 60–70 g (including vegetable 25 g). Carbohydrates: 130–150 g (including simple 0 g). Energy value: 1340-1550 kcal

AUTHOR'S PRESENTATION

Dr. Amin Gasmi is a physiologist and orthomolecular nutritionist. He is currently the president of the Francophone Society of Nutritherapy and Applied Nutrigenetics. He is also the founder and managing editor of the International Journal of Integrative Physiology and Nutritional Sciences. He is a member of several international scientific organizations such as the International Society of Immunonutrition and the International Society of Orthomolecular Medicine. Dr. Gasmi has a multidisciplinary background and had the opportunity to work on several fields such as nutrition sciences, micronutrition, genetics, exercise physiology, applied psychology, physical therapy, physical training, and biochemistry. He has a triple competence of clinician through patients' and athletes' nutritional and physiological care, of scientist through his high quality published books and articles, and of professional trainer through the trainings and lectures he gives to medical doctors, health, and sports professionals.

REFERENCES

Alverdy J. (1994). The effect of nutrition on gastrointestinal barrier function. Semin Respir Infect. 9(4):248-55.

Barnes J. L. (2018). Enteral Nutrients and Gastrointestinal Physiology. J. Infus Nurs. 41(1):35-42.

Bielawska B., Allard J. P. (2017). Parenteral Nutrition and Intestinal Failure. Nutrients. 9(5):466.

Chandler M. (2013). Focus on nutrition: dietary management of gastrointestinal disease. Compend Contin Educ Vet. 35(6): E1-3.

Eswaran S., Farida S., Green J., Miller J. D., Chey W. D. (2017). Nutrition in the management of gastrointestinal diseases and disorders: the evidence for the low FODMAP diet. Curr Opin Pharmacol. 37:151-157.

Gilliland T. M., Villafane-Ferriol N., Shah K. P., Shah R. M., Tran Cao H. S., Massarweh N. N., Silberfein E. J., Choi E. A., Hsu C., McElhany A. L., Barakat O., Fisher W., Van Buren G. (2017). Nutritional and Metabolic Derangements in Pancreatic Cancer and Pancreatic Resection. Nutrients. 9(3):243.

Hasse J. M. (2008). Nutrition in clinical practice. Gastrointestinal disorders and their connections to nutrition. Nutr Clin Pract. 23(3):259.

Jankowski M., Las-Jankowska M., Sousak M., Zegarski W. (2018). Contemporary enteral and parenteral nutrition before surgery for gastrointestinal cancers: a literature review. World J. Surg Oncol. 16(1):94.

Jeejeebhoy K. N. (1998). Nutritional assessment. Gastroenterol Clin North Am. 27(2):347-69.

Le Gall M., Thenet S., Aguanno D., Jarry A. C., Genser L., Ribeiro-Parenti L., Joly F., Ledoux S., Bado A., - Le Beyec J. (2019). Intestinal plasticity in response to nutrition and gastrointestinal surgery. Nutr Rev. 77(3):129-143.

Mandato C., Di Nuzzi A., Vajro P (2017). Nutrition and Liver Disease. Nutrients. 10(1):9.

Merli M., Berzigotti A., Zelber-Sagi S., Dasarathy S., Montagnese S., Genton L., Plauth M., Pares A. (2019). EASL Clinical Practice Guidelines on nutrition in chronic liver disease. J Hepatol. 70(1):172-193.

Morgenroth K., Kozuschek W., Holtz J. (1991). Pancreatitis, Walter de Gruyter, Berlin-New York

Pan L. L., Li J., Shamoon M., Bhatia M., Sun J. (2017). Recent Advances on Nutrition in Treatment of Acute Pancreatitis. Front Immunol. 8:762.

Rasmussen H. H., Irtun O., Olesen S. S., Drewes A. M., Holst M. (2013). Nutrition in chronic pancreatitis. World J. Gastroenterol. 19(42):7267–7275.

Schörghuber M., Fruhwald S. (2018). Effects of enteral nutrition on gastrointestinal function in patients who are critically ill. Lancet Gastroenterol Hepatol. 3(4):281-287.

Shergill R., Syed W., Rizvi S. A., Singh I (2018). Nutritional support in chronic liver disease and cirrhotics. World J Hepatol. 10(10):685–694.

Shu X. L., Kang K., Gu L. J., Zhang Y. S. (2016). Effect of early enteral nutrition on patients with digestive tract surgery: A meta-analysis of randomized controlled trials. Exp Ther Med. 12(4):2136–2144.

Silva M., Gomes S., Peixoto A., Torres-Ramalho P., Cardoso H., Azevedo R., Cunha C., Macedo G. (2015). Nutrition in Chronic Liver Disease. GE Port J Gastroenterol. 22(6):268-276.

Storck L. J., Imoberdorf R., Ballmer P. E. (2019). Nutrition in Gastrointestinal Disease: Liver, Pancreatic, and Inflammatory Bowel Disease. J Clin Med. 25;8(8).

Tomasello G., Mazzola M., Leone A., Sinagra E., Zummo G., Farina F., Damiani P., Cappello F., Gerges Geagea A., Jurjus A., Bou Assi T., Messina M., Carini F. (2016). Nutrition, oxidative stress and intestinal dysbiosis: Influence of diet on gut microbiota in inflammatory bowel diseases. Biomed Pap Med Fac Univ Palacky Olomouc Czech Repub. 160(4):461-466.

Walters J. R. F. (2007). Clinical nutrition in gastrointestinal disease. Gut. 56(10): 1487–1488.

www.ingramcontent.com/pod-product-compliance
Lightning Source LLC
Chambersburg PA
CBHW070311220526
45465CB00004B/1839